SAVING
OUR KIDS

SAVING OUR KIDS

An ER Doc's Common-Sense Solution to the Gun Crisis

Marc Gorelick, MD

President and CEO, Children's Minnesota

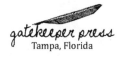
gatekeeper press
Tampa, Florida

SAVING OUR KIDS:

An ER Doc's Common-Sense Solution to the Gun Crisis

Published by Children's Minnesota

Cover Artist: Nikki McComb
McComb is the co-founder and executive director of Art is My Weapon, which uses art as a catalyst for change to creatively address gun violence.

Cover Designer: Dan Sattler-Reimer

Library of Congress Control Number: 2024938073

ISBN (paperback): 9781662930676

DEDICATION

To the thousands of children whose lives have been
affected by gun violence—we owe it to you to do better.

ACKNOWLEDGEMENTS

This book was inspired by my experiences with children who have suffered the effects of gun violence over the years, but it could not have come about without the help of many people to whom I owe a good deal of thanks.

Hillery Shay, who first came up with what seemed like the crazy idea to bring together ideas from my various blog posts into an actual book.

Nick LaFave, whose knowledge of communications and journalism have made this a far more polished product than I could have imagined.

Julianna Olsen, who drafted a good deal of the material and whose gentle yet persistent nudging kept me on track.

The members of the American Academy of Pediatrics Council on Injury, Violence, and Poison Prevention, whose 2022 Policy Statement and Technical Report on Firearm-Related Injuries and Deaths in Children and Youth is a treasure trove of information about this problem and a valuable source for my research.

Drs. Steve Hargarten and Andrew Kiragu, both experts and advocates on gun violence, for their careful review of the manuscript, thoughtful suggestions, and contribution of foreword and afterword.

Dr. Lynn Broaddus, my wife, whose own writing and activism inspire me, whose underlying optimism lifts me up, and whose fundamental belief in people grounds me.

TABLE OF CONTENTS

FOREWORD

Pediatricians have been actively fighting infectious diseases for decades. There is additional advocacy to address heart disease, cancer, and more recently—since the 1960s—motor vehicle crashes. Pediatricians are focused on our nation's most vulnerable: our children.

More and more, physicians, nurses, and other health care providers are engaging these diseases beyond the bedside and within the communities they serve to effectively address disparities and inequities and reduce illnesses and injuries.

More recently, in the past three to four decades, physicians and other healthcare and public health leaders have been actively engaged with another problem: gun violence.

As firearm deaths and injuries have mounted, many more from the broad healthcare and public health communities have declared that gun violence is "in our lane" for prevention and control.

Collectively, we need to address gun violence just like we do all the other diseases of our modern society.

And it's more important than ever. Bullets, from the guns that carry them, are now the leading cause of death in the United States for ages 1–19. Firearms and their bullets have been the leading cause of death for African-American youth for decades.

This timely text, authored by an exemplary physician leader in pediatrics and emergency medicine, is calling for more of us to join in the much-needed clinical care, education, and research to lower this public health burden on our children and teenagers.

In this book, Dr. Marc Gorelick tells his story of engagement and provides the reader with concrete examples of what can and should be done to lower the burden of guns and bullets and help make our communities healthier and safer for everyone.

Dr. Gorelick has documented his personal journey but, more importantly, calls on us who might be on the "sidelines" to join him and others in combatting gun violence in the United States.

His text is filled with important background information and references. Also, as importantly, he suggests ways you and other physicians, health care workers, and public health leaders can work together to make our communities healthier and safer for everyone.

Stephen Hargarten, MD, MPH

Professor, Emergency Medicine

Senior Injury and Policy Advisor, Comprehensive Injury Center

Medical College of Wisconsin

INTRODUCTION

On October 19, 1988, the following letter to the editor appeared in the *Washington Post*:

> *With the campaign against the Maryland gun control law in full swing, one large interest group is notable for its silence— our children. The danger of handguns to children should be self-evident, but the following facts may serve to reinforce the obvious:*
>
> - *Firearms are second only to motor vehicles in causing accidental fatalities among children and adolescents.*
> - *Many of these deaths are attributable to guns in the home. A recent study found that a household gun meant to "protect" the family is actually 18 times more likely to kill a family member than an intruder.*
> - *Carelessness is responsible for a large number of these cases, especially among children. According to a Houston survey, 10% of families reported their guns were always loaded, unlocked, and within reach of a child.*

> • *Easy accessibility of guns is also a major contributor to the shocking epidemic of teenage suicides, currently the third leading cause of death in that age group. More than 2/3 of childhood suicides involve guns.*
>
> *Children cannot lobby, so it remains for those of us who must treat their injuries to make their case for them. Children also cannot vote; fortunately, their parents can.*

That letter was written by me, when I was a second-year pediatric resident in Washington, DC. As you can see, I've been thinking about this problem for a long time! I was moved to write by my firsthand experience caring for young victims of gun violence in our emergency department and intensive care unit (ICU). I wanted to use my voice, my standing as someone who had actually seen what happens when a bullet rips through a child's body, to try to make a difference.

Throughout my thirty-five-year career in pediatrics and pediatric emergency medicine, I have seen far too many of those victims. I carry their stories with me, stories like those I share later in this book. And over that time, unfortunately, the problem has only grown larger and more tragic, while our society's actions to curb the crisis have grown weaker.

Today in America, this is the ugly reality: Nothing kills more children than guns.[1] In 2020, for the first time, gun injuries became the leading cause of death for children. They are shot at home, at school, and in their neighborhoods. There are more guns than ever, with fewer safety measures.

---

1 Goldstick, Jason E., Rebecca M. Cunningham, and Patrick M. Carter, "Current Causes of Death in Children and Adolescents in the United States," *The New England Journal of Medicine* 386, no. 20 (2022): 1955-1956. https://doi.org/10.1056/nejmc2201761.

- In 2021, an average of thirteen children died per day from gunshot wounds.
- Every day of the week, a gun kills a child aged twelve or younger.
- Gun violence has been the number one killer of Black children since at least 1999.[2]

I don't want to overwhelm you with statistics. But I want you to understand how grim the situation is. So here I am again, once more trying to rally those of us who care about kids to stand up for them, to protect those who can't stand up for and protect themselves.

And it keeps getting worse. That is both tragic and unacceptable. I bet most Americans agree. Who can deny that thousands of our kids dying every year in gun-related homicides, suicides, and accidents is simply intolerable? Parents and pediatric professionals, we all want to keep our children safe from harm. We've gone to great lengths in our country to protect them from infectious diseases and car crashes. That's why those are no longer the number one killers of our kids. Now is the time to focus our attention, and especially our action, on this new number one killer.

A Different Way to Think About the Problem

It starts with framing how we think and talk about the problem of gun violence. Too often, we focus solely on the gun. We talk about "gun control" or "gun rights" as if guns exist in a vacuum. As if guns by themselves are out of control or guns themselves have rights. Guns are

---

2 Centers for Disease Control and Prevention. CDC Wonder. (2021).

inanimate objects and, as such, are neither inherently good nor bad. They can have both good effects (venison stew) and bad ones (child in ICU). Cars, drugs, germs like bacteria and viruses, all of these can produce desirable or undesirable outcomes, depending on a lot of other factors. This is the essence of the public health approach to prevention, which I talk much more about later. (Admittedly, in the United States, thanks to the Second Amendment to the Constitution, there are unique considerations when it comes to guns. But the principles of public health still apply.)

You may have heard the expression, attributed to gun rights advocates, "Guns don't kill people. People kill people." Those of us who want to address the issue of gun violence need to acknowledge that, at its root, this is true. It is the combination of guns (or more specifically, bullets), people, and the environment they inhabit that leads to gun violence. Any effort to reduce gun violence must take into account all those factors. Gun violence is a public health problem, one that statistics show is a serious concern and getting worse. Indeed, because the impact is so widespread and continues to grow, it has become a public health *crisis*.

Defining gun violence as a public health crisis for children actually isn't new. The American Academy of Pediatrics (AAP) has been declaring this for decades. The problem is, we're not acting like it. How can we start doing that? By drawing parallels to our most recent major public health crisis, COVID-19, and following the blueprint we created for it, which we can all relate to, to mitigate the gun crisis.

Why I Wrote This Book

Many of us feel helpless—and hopeless—about what guns are doing to our children. I know I sometimes do. Especially after a school shooting like Uvalde. *Good God*, I think, *not again*. We are all horrified. We talk with loved ones about how awful it is. We hear the outcry on TV. We read it in the newspapers. So much anguish, so much handwringing. It's got to end, but how? When?

I don't think we have a motivation problem. For many people, I think it's a "where do we go from here" problem. A "this issue is so stubborn and politically charged, what could I possibly do to change things" problem.

If this is how you feel, I wrote this book for you. If you abhor what you see, but don't know what to do about it, I wrote this book for you. We do not have to accept the status quo. There is a path forward, and throughout the following chapters, I will share that path with you.

Given the lack of action, someone needed to raise awareness of this issue yet again. Someone needed to bring a rational, practical, health-oriented lens to what is, at its root, a health issue. But why me? I've been dealing with this issue for over three decades, both at the bedside and in the boardroom. As a pediatrician, I am both particularly passionate about how guns are harming children and inclined to want to prevent something that is supremely preventable. As a clinical epidemiologist, I know what the public health model is capable of achieving. As a healthcare leader, I see the possibilities and the necessity of systemic change if we are to tackle the scourge of gun violence. Of course, gun violence is a crisis for all Americans, not just children. The total number of gun deaths in our country has been rising every year since 2014.

In 2021, it reached an all-time annual high: 48,000 people of all ages were killed by guns.[3] Sadly, though, I have found that, for too many people, this has become simply background noise. It seems that many only take notice when the victims are kids. So those of us in children's health care need to lead on this issue for the good of all.

In terms of recognizing that gun violence was a problem, it began in the early days of my pediatric residency at what was then known as Children's National Medical Center in Washington, DC, in the late 1980s (1987–1991). I was training to be a pediatric emergency medicine physician. I spent six months of my residency in the emergency department.

At that time, DC was known as the murder capital of the country. The DC murder rate more than doubled from 1987 to 1991.[4] We were the level one trauma center for kids, and we had a lot of gun victims that would come in. Some of them were shot intentionally by others, some of them were shot accidentally by others, some of them shot themselves. But it seemed to me that we had a lot of kids coming in who were being shot. From 1991–1994, I did my fellowship training in pediatric emergency medicine at the Children's Hospital of Philadelphia. I continued to see a fair number of kids with gunshot injuries, and there wasn't much we could do about it.

As a pediatrician, I was primed to place a lot of emphasis on prevention—disease prevention and injury prevention. We gave vaccines

---

3 John Gramlich, "What the data says about gun deaths in the U.S.," *Pew Research Center*, April 26, 2023, https://www.pewresearch.org/short-reads/2023/04/26/what-the-data-says-about-gun-deaths-in-the-u-s/.

4 "District of Columbia Crime Rates 1960 to 2019," Disaster Center, https://disaster-center.com/crime/dccrime.htm.

and advised on hygiene to prevent infections. We promoted car seats and car safety, playground safety, sports equipment improvements, and so on. We counseled families during clinic and emergency department visits, and we advocated for policies to keep kids safe and healthy.

From what I saw in my practice, gun violence seemed to be ripe for the same kinds of preventions. The way I approached it at first was individual advocacy: writing to legislators and that kind of thing. I also became involved with the American Academy of Pediatrics, the leading advocacy organization for children's health and longtime proponents of measures to reduce harm from guns to children, eventually becoming Chair of the AAP's Section on Emergency Medicine. In the early '90s, it seemed like policy advocacy could yield results: the Brady Bill in 1993, an assault weapons ban in 1994 at the federal level, and a variety of state and local legislation in different parts of the country were huge steps in reducing the risk to kids (and others) from gun violence.

These were important measures, and as I discuss later, research shows that they saved lives, but over time, the appetite for policy solutions waned. It appeared the discussion became not about gun violence but about guns. By the time the assault weapons ban expired in 2004, it couldn't get renewed.

As I moved on in my career into increasing leadership roles, I felt like I had both the ability and the obligation to do more to raise awareness and promote solutions. First, I engaged in what I call "low-key advocacy." I would take people on tours through the emergency department as part of my role as the department chief. I would always show them the trauma room and talk to them about gunshot victims, even though that wasn't by any stretch of the imagination most of the patients we saw. But it was something I was able to talk about with people who might be in a position to care, to do something: board members, donors, community leaders. I wanted to help them understand what it's like to see that kind of patient.

Then, with a hospital leadership role, I was in even more of a position to drive a change. Nobody cared about what Dr. Marc Gorelick had to say, but they might care about what the chief operating officer of a major children's hospital had to say. That's when I started writing about it and feeling I could use my position to drive some change. It was not because I was any more horrified than I'd been twenty years earlier—that's not possible—but because I had an opportunity to make sure others were as horrified as I was. Horrified enough to want to make a difference.

Over my career, I've seen other health crises get better. I've seen diseases that used to fill up our hospital wards basically disappear because we have vaccines for them. For example, there's a particular kind of infection that affects infants. It's called *Haemophilus influenza* type b or Hib. We routinely saw kids come into the hospital with serious infections, meningitis, and other infections. A vaccine came out shortly after I was a resident, and it's rare to see that anymore.

Even something as common as rotavirus, which causes diarrheal illness, has a vaccine now. It greatly reduced the severity of illness, with many fewer hospitalizations than there were fifteen to twenty years ago. For many types of injuries, those rates have gone down, too. If you look at pediatric fatalities from car crashes, those have been going steadily down because of laws, technology, and safety improvements.

I've seen all those other things get better, but gun violence is not. Why is it getting worse when we've made progress with so many other health threats? It doesn't need to be this way. We can do better.

Who This Book Is For

When we frame the issue of guns as a public health threat to children, we place it firmly in the purview of everyone who cares about kids' health: parents and families and other caregivers, health care professionals, educators, policymakers, children themselves, and everyone else who is devoted to the wellbeing of young people. This is an enormous group. Together, we can make a resounding change. Indeed, both moms and pediatricians have been at the forefront of advancing injury control. We need to keep at it.

Part of my goal with this book is to be of service to anyone who wants to speak on this issue in a public health light. So when they are talking to their legislator who is a big gun advocate, they can talk about gun violence not as a Second Amendment issue but as a public health issue. They can say, "I'm a pediatrician." Or "I'm a parent." "I don't know anything about constitutional law, but I do know about kids' health."

That's how I hope this book will make a difference. This is a really important, really charged issue. How can we do a better job of addressing it? I often hear from people that they're scared to bring up the issue of gun safety. They don't know what to say; they're afraid it's going to be too controversial, too polarizing.

From my perspective as a father and a doctor, I present this book to you as a roadmap to a better way of thinking and talking about the problem of gun violence that will lead to change. I hope it will galvanize you to take action. I want to enlist all of you in addressing the gun crisis as vigorously as we addressed COVID-19 so that, next year and every year after that, guns will no longer pose a significant threat to our children's lives.

CHAPTER 1

WHAT IS THE PROBLEM?

This is not the same crisis we had twenty or even ten years ago. What was a serious problem when I was going through my medical training has now become a public health emergency. Everyone who cares for kids—healthcare workers, parents, and grandparents—needs to be engaged in addressing gun violence like never before because kids are dying like never before.

Recent studies in *Pediatrics* and the *New England Journal of Medicine* show that, thanks to a sharp decline in deaths from motor vehicle crashes and an increase in gun deaths (especially suicide), gun violence became the leading cause of death for all US youth aged 0–19 in 2020. **THE** leading cause of death. For kids. More than childhood cancer, drowning, or poisoning combined. When I first saw those studies, I couldn't believe what I was reading. Whenever I tell someone that guns are now the leading cause of death for kids, they can't believe it either. Sadly, this is the reality.

The numbers below come from the Centers for Disease Control (CDC) and its Web-based Injury Statistics Query and Reporting System (WISQARS™). As you'll see in the table below, the data is not comprehensive, but there's enough to tell a distressing story.

Estimated Gunshot-Related Injuries and Deaths 2012–2021, United States[1]
1 to 19-year-olds (all demographics)

CAUSE	UNINTENTIONAL	VIOLENCE-RELATED	SELF-HARM	ALL
FATAL	1200	19,587	11,563	32,866
NON-FATAL	29,751	139,841	N/A*	174,005
TOTAL	30,951	159,428	11,563	206,871

*Not available: injury estimate is not shown because it is
unstable due to small sample size and/or CV > 30%.*

From 2012–2021, nearly 33,000 children aged 1–19 years died from firearm injuries. (No, that is not a typo.) That means nine young people died every single day over the course of ten years. They are shot at home, at school, and in their neighborhoods. Firearms, now the leading cause of death in childhood, account for 24% of all deaths among children and adolescents. As you can see in the table, for each death from gun violence, there are at least five non-lethal injuries. (I say at least five because there are not great data on non-fatal injuries due to self-harm.) From 2012 to 2021, more than 200,000 American kids suffered gunshot injuries.

In 2021 alone, more than 29,000 children (aged 1-19) were treated for (lethal and non-lethal) gunshot injuries in emergency rooms across the United States. Just ten years earlier, that number was around 15,000. The rate of non-fatal firearm injuries for kids per 100,000 people increased by 96%, while the fatal injury rate rose by 77%.

---

1 Centers for Disease Control and Prevention. CDC WISQARS (2012 – 2021).

Mass shootings are horrible, and they make for sensational headlines, but they're not even close to the biggest part of the problem when it comes to gun violence. Some of these injuries are accidental, but for 10–14-year-olds, half are self-inflicted, while almost one-third of deaths in teens are suicide. (Note that guns are not the most common method of self-harm in youth, just the most lethal.) And of the homicides, the vast majority are due to domestic violence or interpersonal disputes, not a stranger coming into their school.

Disparities in Firearm Deaths

The fact that firearm injuries are now the leading cause of death in children has generated some media attention. While I am grateful for the increased focus on the problem, I have mixed feelings. After all, firearm injury has been the leading cause of death for Black youth since at least 1999.

Yes, firearm injury and death are another part of American society rife with disparities. Here are just a few recent examples:

- Black youth are eleven times more likely to die from a firearm homicide than White youth.[2]
- The rate of firearm suicide is highest among American Indian and Alaska Native youth.[3]
- The firearm mortality rate due to legal intervention in adolescents (up to age seventeen) is six times higher for Blacks and almost three times higher for Hispanic adolescents compared with Whites.[4]

---

2 Bailey K. Roberts et al., "Trends and Disparities in Firearm Deaths Among Children," *Pediatrics* 152, no. 3 (2023): 4, https://doi.org/10.1542/peds.2023-061296.

3 Roberts et al., "Trends and Disparities,"

4 Roberts et al., "Trends and Disparities,"

Why are young people of color more impacted by gun violence than their White counterparts? It's not because they are inherently more prone to violence or suicide. It's because they often grow up in communities greatly impacted by structural racism and historical inequities, communities that lack investment, opportunity, and hope.

The Johns Hopkins Center for Gun Violence Solutions identifies these six root causes of gun violence in communities of color:[5]

- Income inequality
- Poverty
- Underfunded public housing
- Under-resourced public services
- Underperforming schools
- Lack of opportunity and perceptions of hopelessness
- Easy access to firearms by high-risk people

The factors that lead a young person to experience gun violence are complex, as I discuss in Chapter 3. But for many young people of color, economic and social disadvantages only increase their chances.

All of the statistics we have just reviewed are shocking. They are heartbreaking. But the fact is, they are not statistics. These are individuals. Children. Children like the little girl I once took care of who was hit by a stray bullet while riding her bike, or the thirteen-year-old who mutilated herself while trying to take her own life with her father's

---

5 "The Root Causes of Gun Violence," *The Educational Fund to Stop Gun Violence*, March 2020, https://efsgv.org/wp-content/uploads/2020/03/EFSGV-The-Root-Causes-ofGun-Violence-March-2020.pdf.

gun, or the children in the classrooms in Sandy Hook and Parkview and Uvalde. Too many children. Children who we are supposed to keep safe.

A recent Kaiser Family Foundation survey revealed the extent to which gun violence has become part of routine life in this country, especially for people of color.[6] More than half (54%) of all Americans report having been personally affected by gun violence, either personally threatened, witnessing a shooting, or having a family member killed by a gun. One in three Black adults has had a family member killed by gun violence compared with 17% of Whites. This is not okay.

Why Is This Happening?

Undoubtedly there are several factors contributing to the rising gun death rate for children. One clear factor, though, is the sheer number of guns. Gun sales in the US increased by 76% from 2011-2021.[7] According to reporting in the *New York Times*, while the US has just 4.4% of the world's population, it has 42% of the world's guns and nearly 90% of the firearm deaths.[8] With ninety guns per one hundred members of the population, per capita gun ownership is nearly twice that of the next highest country (Yemen) and about three times that

---

6 Shannon Schumacher et al., "Americans' Experience With Gun-Related Violence, Injuries, And Deaths," *Kaiser Family Foundation*, April 11, 2023, https://www.kff.org/other/poll-finding/americansexperiences-with-gun-related-violence-injuries-and-deaths/.

7 Rob Gabriele, "Gun Sales in the U.S.:2024 Statistics," *SafeHome.org*, June 17,2024, https://www.safehome.org/data/firearms-guns-statistics/.

8 Max Fisher and Josh Keller, "Why Does the U.S. Have So Many Mass Shootings? Research Is Clear: Guns," *The New York Times*, November 7, 2017, https://www.nytimes.com/2017/11/07/world/americas/mass-shootings-us-international.html?smid=url-share.

of the next closest wealthy countries, Canada and France. But even this comparison is misleading, as a higher proportion of guns in the US are handguns (which are far more likely to be involved in gun-related deaths). In the US, 47% of guns are handguns vs. 9% in Canada.

Looking specifically at mass shootings, a University of Alabama researcher found that gun ownership rate was the strongest predictor of mass shooting rates across countries after adjusting for demographics, other violent crime rates, and mental illness (using suicide rates as an indicator).[9]

Even within our own country, studies have shown that the number of guns correlates with rates of suicide, homicide, and accidental firearm injury and death. For example, in 2021, researchers found that a ten-percentage point increase in state gun ownership rate is associated with a 27% increase in the youth suicide rate.[10]

Several other factors appear to be salient in the increase in child gun deaths. Not only are there more guns, but with technology constantly evolving, they have become more lethal. The increased rate of mental illness in children and youth is a likely factor specifically in gun suicide. And COVID-19 appears to only have exacerbated the already existing mental health crisis among our youth. It's too early to know the full impact of COVID-19, but during the pandemic, gun suicide deaths rose among young people aged 10–19.

---

9 "Adam Lankford, "Public Mass Shooters and Firearms: A Cross-National Study of 171 Countries," *Violence and Victims* 31, no. 2 (2016): 192, https://doi.org/10.1891/0886-6708.VV-D-15-00093.

10 Anita Knopov et al., "Household Gun Ownership and Youth Suicide Rates at the State Level, 2005-2015," *American Journal of Preventative Medicine,* 56, no. 3 (2019): 339, https://doi.org/10.1016/j.amepre.2018.10.027.

Finally, we must acknowledge that the regulatory climate has changed, especially since the Heller decision by the Supreme Court in 2008. All of these are discussed in more detail in Chapter 3.

Guns vs. Gun Violence

Some would argue that guns are a partisan issue. I would counter that *guns* have become a partisan issue but gun *violence* need not be. The approach to gun violence is by definition a political issue, as is any public health threat, because it must be addressed in part through good public policies. But public health can and should be addressed in a bi-partisan—or ideally, non-partisan—way.

For example, our country's response to COVID-19 wasn't perfect. But before the introduction of vaccines, when the virus posed the biggest danger, Americans were mostly united in a common purpose: taking health precautions, enacting policies, and developing counter-measures to minimize sickness and death. And studies show that those actions undoubtedly saved many lives. When COVID-19 became a partisan issue, progress faltered. But when we focus on the policies, not on the people or parties promoting them, we have shown that progress is possible.

Many more kids have died from gun violence than from COVID-19. Since early 2020, COVID-19 has taken the lives of more than 1,800 children. In that same time, more than 15,000 children have died from gunshots. If we approach the gun violence crisis with lessons learned during the COVID-19 pandemic, we can save children's lives. Defining guns as a public health, not a partisan, issue leads us to solutions, just as it did for smoking, car crashes, and COVID-19.

CHAPTER 2

WHAT GUNS DO

Too often, gun violence feels like an abstraction. For many of us, knowledge about gun violence comes only through the media. We read the statistics, and they are just numbers; we hear the intellectual arguments, and they come across as coolly rational. As Stalin said, "One death is a tragedy; a million deaths is a statistic." It seems it's only when there is a Sandy Hook or a Uvalde that we get hit in the gut with *Oh, my God, this is what we're talking about: dead kids.*

To me, as a pediatric emergency medicine physician, it's never been an abstraction. It's something I dealt with and saw, far too many times and in a raw and real way. Duty compelled me to manage each gunshot victim with composure, but it was never easy. It sounds really shocking to find out there's a six-year-old with a gunshot who's coming in, and you would typically think, *Oh, my gosh, no,* but you quickly learn not to be shocked by it—or rather, to put off the shock. Because you're running a team, you have to make sure that you have the people, the equipment, and most importantly, the focus to take care of that patient. You learn to defer your personal reaction in the interest of getting mobilized.

Defer but not deflect. I've always said, if anybody ever gets used to this, they probably should stop doing it. It's not about getting used to it. It's about adapting to it. Every time I've taken care of somebody with a serious gunshot injury, I've cried. But I do it later. I do it when we're done, when the child who's been shot doesn't need me to keep it together anymore. And that's when I let myself be shocked and grieve.

What Do Guns Do to a Child's Body?

In my nearly twenty-five years as a pediatric emergency physician, I have seen shattered bodies like these:

- A teenage boy bleeding to death after he was shot by a friend following an argument over a phone, his limbs swollen grotesquely from the fluid we pumped into his body in a desperate attempt to keep up with the blood pouring from the wounds in his chest and belly, his color fading, and the bleeding eventually stopping when his heart stopped.

- A seven-year-old girl with pieces of her shattered femur sticking through her skin after a stray bullet went through her leg while she was riding her bike.

- A thirteen-year-old girl who blew off most of her face when she tried to kill herself with her father's shotgun, one eye gone and the other dangling, crying for her parents through the half of her mouth that remained.

This is what guns do.

We all have an image of what COVID-19 does to a person's body. So many pictures and videos of unconscious people, alone in the hospital, hooked up to ventilators for weeks, months on end. Heart-breaking. Did it motivate you to wear a mask or get a vaccine? In the same vein, what about guns? What do they do to a child's body? I wonder, if more people saw it firsthand, the way I have—small, innocent human beings, mutilated and destroyed—would they be shocked into action?

When Mamie Till's son Emmett was brutally tortured and lynched in Mississippi in 1955, she insisted that the world needed to see what she saw. His battered corpse was on view in an open-casket funeral attended by hundreds and shown in newspapers around the world. Racial violence was no longer an abstraction that could be glossed over. It was a raw, ugly reality not only to its victims but to the entire public. It was a key moment in spurring the civil rights movement.

Sadly, some gun deaths I watched didn't even make the news. After all, there isn't enough room in the papers to report on every person felled by a gun. But crime still sells, and there are plenty of media items about gun violence. In 2015, in the wake of recent mass shootings, the *New York Times* ran its first front-page editorial in almost a century.

That won't do it. People don't need to be convinced, as most of them say they agree something needs to be done; they need to be shocked out of complacency. Is it time to do what Mamie Till did? Is it time to stop showing photos of the perpetrators or grainy school pictures of the victims and show the graphic, gruesome results instead? That may be too much. At the very least, those like me who have seen the carnage need to share our stories and bear witness. Everyone needs to know what guns really do.

The Survivors

It's hard to fathom how an object we can hold in the palm of our hand can have such a powerful impact on our children. We've talked about the damage guns have on a child's body and how they take children's lives. What about the kids who experience gun violence and survive?

Every day in the United States, children are injured by guns. They witness shootings, hear gunshots fired, hear about gun violence in the news and in their communities, and lose loved ones to guns. For some kids, they experience all these traumatic events; gun violence is a routine part of their lives.

As you can imagine, these events deeply impact children. Whether seen, heard, or experienced in some other way, gun violence affects children's physical and psychological health. We can't ignore these negative health effects when we consider the public health toll guns have on our kids.

Unfortunately, while the numbers of child deaths from guns are well-documented, the physical, mental, and emotional consequences of gun violence on children are not. Part of the reason may be that these impacts are harder to track and quantify than deaths. But there's also a dearth of research due to a legal provision that, since 1996, has hampered the study of the public health effects of guns.

This provision is called the Dickey Amendment. It says, "None of the funds made available for injury prevention and control at the Centers for Disease Control and Prevention (CDC) may be used to advocate or promote gun control." To avoid violating this amendment and possible repercussions, the CDC has steered clear of gun violence research. In the last few years, this chill has started to warm, and in 2018, Congress clarified that the amendment (which is still in effect) does *not* prohibit funding of research on gun violence.

Yet gun research remains woefully underfunded compared with the public health impact gun violence has. For example, in 2020, approximately $6 billion of federal funding went to cancer research, including $250 million for childhood cancer (which causes fewer than 2,000 deaths per year),[1] compared to just $25 million for gun violence, which caused almost 5,000 child deaths in 2021.[2] It is estimated that federal investment in gun research equates to $57 for each firearm-related death compared to nearly $3,000 per death from cancer and $6,500 per death from lung disease.[3] While we are starting to see more studies on the public health effects of guns, it will be some time before we have a comprehensive body of research.

Nevertheless, there is evidence showing that when children witness or experience gun violence, it can have long-lasting physical and psychological consequences. These consequences are very much a part of the equation when we're considering the public health risks guns have for children.

---

1 "2023 NCI Budget Fact Book – Research Funding – NCI," *National Cancer Institute,* June 20, 2024, https://www.cancer.gov/types/childhood-cancers/child-adolescent-cancers-fact-sheet#:~:text=In%202021%2C%20it%20is%20estimated,of%20the%20disease%20(1).

2 "Research Funding," *Everytown for Gun Safety Action Fund,* https://everytownresearch.org/issue/research-funding/.

3 "Research Funding," Giffords: *Courage to Fight Gun Violence,* https://giffords.org/issues/research-funding/.

Physical Effects

In 2020, more than 24,000 kids were injured by a gun and survived.[4] Over a few years, the number of young gunshot survivors adds up quickly. As noted in the prior chapter, for every child aged 1–19 who is killed by a gun, there are five or six who are injured seriously enough to go to the emergency department. (If you need another indication of how deadly guns are, consider that, for non-gun injuries in this age group, the ratio of non-fatal to fatal injuries is 452.)

Now, many of these injuries are relatively minor, and the child will recover without any significant physical sequelae. In other cases, there is permanent, often debilitating damage. The young girl I mentioned above, who attempted to take her own life, was left blind and disfigured. Nearly all my colleagues have anecdotes similar to mine. We don't have any good data on long-term physical disability related to pediatric gun injury, though a 2020 study of young adults with non-fatal gunshot wounds showed worse physical health and physical functioning and greater pain intensity than a comparable non-injured group. On the other hand, we are starting to get a clear picture of the mental health consequences for kids. It is not a pretty picture.

Psychological Effects

Recently, I was participating in a community bike ride for sickle cell disease. I was talking with a young woman, a sickle cell patient, who was also participating. She's a teacher in the Minneapolis Public

---

4 "WISQARS Explore Fatal and Nonfatal Data." n.d. Centers for Disease Control and Prevention. https://wisqars.cdc.gov/explore/?o=MORT&y1=2018&y2=2018&g=00&t=0&i=2&m=20890&d=&s=0&r=0&me=0&ry=0&yp=65&e=0&a=custom&a1=1&a2=19&g1=0&g2=199.

Schools. We were riding along, and when we got to a particular corner, she said, "My students saw somebody shot on this corner. And they've been suffering really bad." It just came up in conversation; this is the corner where her students saw somebody get shot, and they're really struggling with it. I'm not sure if I was more shocked by the fact that we were riding past the site where this had happened or the matter-of-fact way she related the story to me.

The fact is, bullets can shatter not just the body but also the psyche. Mental health is another crisis our young people are facing, and gun violence is one contributing factor. When you look at the list of traumatic life events (like death of a child or parent) that cause physical and mental health problems, experiencing or witnessing violence is fairly high up on the list. Researchers have studied the psychological effects of violence on children in general, but little data exists on solely the effects of gun violence.

A 2009 meta-analysis of 114 published studies of the effects of community violence (not specifically gun violence) on children and adolescents concluded that being a direct victim of community violence and witnessing and even hearing about violence in their community was correlated with a number of adverse mental health outcomes.[5] Among younger children, internalizing symptoms such as withdrawal, depression, and anxiety were more common, while adolescents were more likely to exhibit acting out and aggressive behavior. Symptoms of

---

5 Patrick J. Folwer et al., "Community violence: A meta-analysis on the effect of exposure and mental health outcomes of children and adolescents," *Development and Psychopathology* 21, no. 1 (2009): 227-259, https://doi.org/10.1017/s0954579409000145.

posttraumatic stress and disruption of relationships are also associated with exposure to violence.

More specific to the issue of firearms, studies have found similar patterns of psychological harm. Much of the research has focused on children and youth in urban areas, but this is not an isolated issue. In 2019, a group of researchers published a study titled "Gun Violence Exposure and Posttraumatic Symptoms Among Children and Youth."[6] The researchers surveyed, either directly or through their parents, more than 600 demographically diverse children (aged 2–17) from Boston, Philadelphia, and rural Tennessee. The survey included questions on various exposures to gun violence: direct exposure, witnessing, and hearing.

Among the researchers' findings:

- Hearing guns fired in public places was the most common type of reported exposure and was experienced by almost 50% of youth 10–17 years of age and 28% of 2–9-year-olds in this sample.

- Among 2–9-year-olds, both witnessing gun violence and hearing gunshots in public were significantly related to levels of posttraumatic symptoms, independent of demographic factors; direct gun violence was not considered given the small number of cases in this age group.

- The level of threat does not need to be especially serious to create significant distress in younger children.

6 Heather A. Turner et al., "Gun Violence Exposure and Posttraumatic Symptoms Among Children and Youth," *Journal of Traumatic Stress* 32, no. 6 (2019): 881-889, https://doi.org/10.1002/ jts.22466.

- Among 10–17-year-olds, both direct gun violence exposure and witnessing gun violence were significantly related to posttraumatic symptoms, after controlling for demographic variables.

Financial Cost

We've examined the enormous physical and psychological toll of gun violence on children. The impact on their lives and health is by far the biggest, most heart-wrenching toll. But there's another toll. What does all of their physical and emotional trauma cost us in dollars?

I have a unique perspective on the issue of gun violence because of my training as an emergency physician but also as a clinical epidemiologist and healthcare leader. The fact is there's a huge cost in helping kids who have been shot. To some, that will sound insensitive and crass. For others, it may be a persuasive argument. Regardless of whether we want to talk about it or not, it has a huge negative impact on American society.

Approximating the financial impact of a public health crisis of any kind is challenging. There are direct healthcare costs, which are relatively easy to estimate, but even this can be fraught. You need to account for the immediate treatment of the gun injury but also the costs of follow-up and managing long-term physical consequences. Any estimate would also need to consider the costs of caring for the psychological sequelae as well, which would necessarily be more imprecise given the nature of the available data.

Then there are many types of indirect costs to society. In the case of firearm fatalities, there is the cost of the lost years of productive life;

one can similarly estimate the value of lost quality-adjusted years due to long-term disability. There are also the costs of managing the threat of gun violence, everything from tangible risk reduction measures, such as metal detectors and vehicle escorts, to criminal investigations and incarceration.

With all these caveats, a recent estimate from Everytown for Gun Safety found an annual national economic cost of $557 billion due to gun violence, equivalent to 2.6% of US GDP. That is $1.53 billion *every single day*.[7] This included:

- $7.8 million each day in medical costs
- $149 million each day due to lost productivity
- $30 million each day in police and criminal justice costs
- $1.34 billion each day in quality-of-life costs

For context, the authors of that report point out that $557 billion is five times the budget for the Department of Education.

Data from the CDC allow us to come up with an estimate of the societal cost of gun violence specifically for kids. In 2020, the total cost just of fatal gun violence for children nineteen and under was $64.7 billion dollars.[8] (I was unable to find good data available estimating the cost of non-fatal firearm injury specifically in kids, so that estimate is,

---

7 "The Economic Cost of Gun Violence," *Everytown for Gun Safety Action Fund,* July 19, 2022, https://everytownresearch.org/report/the-economic-cost-of-gun-violence/.

8 "WISQARS Cost of Injury." n.d. Centers for Disease Control and Prevention. https://wisqars. cdc.gov/cost/?y=2021&o=MORT&i=0&m=20890&g=00&s=0&u=TOTAL&t=-COMBO&t=M ED&t=VPSL&a=custom&g1=0&g2=199&a1=1&a2=19&r1=MECH&r2=INTENT&r3=NONE &r4=NONE&c1=NONE&c2=NONE.

of course, a bare minimum.) Similar to the numbers above, the large majority of that cost is due to the wasteful loss of human life.

Mangled bodies, damaged psyches, shattered families and communities, billions of wasted dollars: this is what guns do.

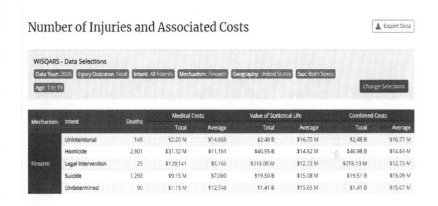

Number of Injuries and Associated Costs

WISQARS - Data Selections

Data Year: 2020 Injury Outcome: Fatal Intent: All Intents Mechanism: Firearm Geography: United States Sex: Both Sexes
Age: 1 to 19

Mechanism	Intent	Deaths	Medical Costs		Value of Statistical Life		Combined Costs	
			Total	Average	Total	Average	Total	Average
Firearm	Unintentional	148	$2.20 M	$14,888	$2.48 B	$16.75 M	$2.48 B	$16.77 M
	Homicide	2,801	$31.32 M	$11,181	$40.95 B	$14.62 M	$40.98 B	$14.63 M
	Legal Intervention	25	$129,141	$5,166	$318.00 M	$12.72 M	$318.13 M	$12.73 M
	Suicide	1,293	$9.15 M	$7,080	$19.50 B	$15.08 M	$19.51 B	$15.09 M
	Undetermined	90	$1.15 M	$12,748	$1.41 B	$15.65 M	$1.41 B	$15.67 M

CHAPTER 3

PUBLIC HEALTH, NOT PARTISAN WARFARE

It does not matter whether we believe that guns kill people or that people kill people with guns—the result is the same: a public health crisis.

—THE EDITORS OF THE ANNALS OF INTERNAL MEDICINE

Few issues in America have become more polarizing than guns. On one end of the spectrum, you have Second Amendment hardliners who bristle at any hint that gun ownership will be curtailed or regulated in any way. On the opposite side are people who want all guns outlawed. There's not even agreement on how to label it and talk about it, "gun control" vs. "gun safety."

Most Americans fall between these two extremes, and historically, there has been less of a chasm. For example, until the 1970s, the National Rifle Association (NRA) supported a variety of federal legislation regulating the sale and possession of firearms. As with so many other matters with public policy implications, when addressing gun violence becomes overly partisan, it leads down a dead-end road.

We need a better way. We must reframe what gun violence is and examine it in a new light so we can more clearly see how to prevent it. Where can we find common ground?

We can find it in science. More specifically, we can find it in public health.

We start with the fact that gun violence is a disease, a matter of public health. For many reasons, which we'll discuss in this chapter, considering gun violence as a disease is not a very big leap. To solve it, we must approach gun violence like other public health threats we've faced. Like other public health problems, there is by necessity an element of public policy that is part of the solution. So in that sense, gun violence is a *political* issue, but it need not be a *partisan* issue.

How is gun violence a disease? In simple terms, Merriam-Webster defines disease as "a condition of the living animal or...one of its parts that impairs normal functioning and is typically manifested by distinguishing signs and symptoms." When we breathe in the SARS-CoV-2 coronavirus, it causes damage that leads to symptoms of COVID-19. When cigarette smoke enters our lungs, it causes damage that produces cancer and its myriad effects. When a bullet enters a human body, the energy of that bullet damages the structure and functioning of the tissues, just as a germ or toxin does. If COVID-19 is a disease, if cancer is a disease, then gun injury is also a disease.

Epidemic Proportions

In keeping with the convention of considering gun violence a disease, it's fair to say that, over the last few years, this disease has reached epidemic proportions for children.

According to the Centers for Disease Control and Prevention, "Epidemic refers to an increase, often sudden, in the number of cases of a disease above what is normally expected in that population in that area."

I challenge you to conduct a brief experiment. Ask a handful of people what they think is the number one killer of kids in our country. You'll get a variety of answers: infection, cancer, car crashes, and drowning are common responses. I'll bet very few, if any, will answer that guns are the number one killer of kids.

From 1999 through 2013, gun deaths among children (aged 1–19) generally trended downward.[1] In 2014, about 2,500 kids died from gun violence, and the numbers began to rise from there.

In 2021, the most recent year we have data for, guns killed more than 4,700 children; 685 more kids died from guns that year than from motor vehicle crashes, making guns, for the second year in a row, the number one killer of kids. The increase is seen in both teens and younger kids, in both urban and rural areas, among kids of all races. (By the way, the number one killer of adults is heart disease. In 2021, gun violence didn't break the top ten causes of death for adults.)

---

1 Goldstick et al., "Current Causes of Death," 1955.

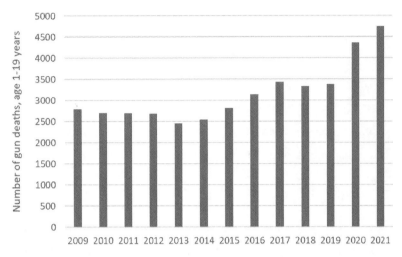

Source: WISQARS ™. Data reflects homicide, suicide, and unintentional deaths.

That sure looks like an epidemic to me.

Think about that. Guns are the number one killer of kids. There is no telethon dedicated to eradicating gun violence. There are no change boxes at cash registers to raise money to help kids who have been shot. Guns kill more kids than cancer, diabetes, and heart disease. Yet of the fifty largest disease foundations devoted to kids' illnesses, not one is for gun violence.

As shocking as this is, it is an unfortunate fact that guns have been the leading cause of death for Black kids for many years. Rates of gun death from both intentional and accidental causes remain substantially higher for Black and other youth of color, while gun suicide rates have historically been highest among White youth. But in 2022, for the first time, the gun suicide rate among Black youth (aged 10–19) eclipsed the rate among White youth (aged 10–19).[2] This is another sobering example of the kind of health disparities arising from structural racism.

Biopsychosocial Public Health Model

Disease doesn't just happen randomly. Some disease agents are virulent, while others are more innocuous. Individuals and populations differ in their susceptibility to diseases. To identify the causes and contributing factors of disease, understand why it spreads, and ultimately prevent it, public health experts have developed a model called the public health triad. The public health triad is like a three-legged stool. It has three equally important factors that must be present for a disease to spread: an external agent, a susceptible host, and an environment that brings the host and agent together.

Originally used to explain infectious diseases, the model has been adopted to investigate a variety of chronic conditions and injuries. If we're talking about an infectious disease, the external agent would be a germ, like the COVID-19 virus. The susceptible host would be the person who contracts the germ, COVID-19, and then becomes impaired with symptoms like coughing, aches, and fatigue. The environment is wherever the susceptible host, or person, came in contact with the external agent, COVID-19. The environment could be a family gathering where someone coughed the COVID-19 germ into the air, and a susceptible host, another person, breathed in the virus and became impaired with symptoms over the following days.

---

2 "CDC Provisional Data: Gun Suicides Reach All-time High in 2022, Gun Homicides Down Slightly from 2021," *Johns Hopkins Bloomberg School of Public Health,* July 27, 2023, https://publichealth.jhu.edu/center-for-gun-violence-solutions/2023/cdc-provisional-data-gun-suicides-reach-all-time-high-in-2022-gun-homicides-down-slightly-from-2021.

For chronic illnesses and injuries, it is helpful to modify that public health model in a way that recognizes explicitly that behavioral factors are a critical influence on susceptibility. The biopsychosocial model of disease, first introduced by physician and psychoanalyst George Engel in 1977, can be used to study diseases at both the individual and the population levels. Like the public health triad, there are three components: physical, or biological; psychological, or behavioral; and social, or environmental.

For COVID-19, the physical factors would include not only the coronavirus itself—the contagiousness and pathogenicity of the strain, for example—but also whether a person has other underlying health risks or immunity from a vaccine or prior infection. The behavioral factors might include what a person did or didn't do to protect or expose themselves to COVID-19, such as participating in social distancing, handwashing, or wearing a mask. The social factors relevant to the spread of COVID-19 include whether businesses are open or masks or vaccines are required.

Gun violence fits neatly into the commonly used model of the public health triad or biopsychosocial model. Let's examine this in more detail.

Biological Contributors to Child Gun Deaths

The biological, or physical, agent of disease with gun violence is actually the bullet. A bullet fired from a gun carries a tremendous amount of kinetic energy. When the bullet enters a human body, that energy is transferred to the body's tissues in the form of shock waves that spread through those tissues, creating immense damage in its wake. As with other diseases, the characteristics of the physical agent are an important factor in the severity of the damage caused. The weight, caliber, shape, and composition of the bullet, for example, are factors in their lethality. Guns vary in the velocity with which bullets are fired, depending on the caliber, barrel length, and cartridge power. Of course, the gun's capacity and ability to fire repeatedly also affect its virulence, as multiple bullets will cause more damage than one. A variety of features, such as safeties, locks, and fingerprint recognition technology, can influence the ability of the gun to cause harm.

As we saw in Chapter 1, the physical agents of gun injury have become more lethal in recent years. Semi-automatic guns, such as the AR-15, can fire up to sixty rounds per minute; with high-capacity magazines containing upward of ten rounds each that are changeable in just a few seconds, assault rifles can deliver an immense number of bullets in a very brief period of time. Assault weapons also release bullets at a greater velocity than other guns. This makes them deadlier since the damage caused is related to the kinetic energy of the bullet, which is proportional to the square of its velocity.

In addition, multiple gunshot wounds are more likely to be fatal than single gunshot wounds, and the proportion of victims with multiple gunshot wounds has increased over the past twenty years. At the same time that guns have become more deadly, so has ammunition. The caliber of bullets most sold and used in the US has increased in recent years, and research has shown that larger (higher caliber) bullets are more likely to cause lethal injury. Moreover, smaller guns that are easier to carry and conceal are able to fire larger bullets than in the past. The combination of higher velocity and higher caliber bullets has led to higher rates of death and more severe injuries.

Psychological/Behavioral Contributors to Child Gun Deaths

It is a common trope to say, "Guns don't kill people; people kill people." Of course, this is both true and silly. People kill people with guns. However, it does underscore the second element of the biopsychosocial model, the behavioral element. When it comes to explaining the increase in gun deaths among children, there is a good deal of speculation but little firm evidence on what the key behavioral factors are.

Mental health is often suggested as a blanket factor in gun violence. There is a component of this that is probably true, but it's more complex than that. There has certainly been an alarming increase in the rate of mental illness among kids and youth that has correlated with the increase in firearm fatalities. This is almost certainly an important factor in the increase in gun suicides, which accounted for 35% of child and youth firearm deaths between 2011 and 2020. From 2009 to 2016, the prevalence of depression among American high school students increased by 50%;[3] preliminary data suggest a much steeper increase since 2020. From 2011 to 2021, a study showed that, among high school youth, the rates of suicidal thoughts, suicidal planning, and suicide attempts all increased.[4]

---

3 Sylia Wilson and Nathalie M. Dumornay, "Rising Rates of Adolescent Depression in the United States: Challenges and Opportunities in the 2020s," *Journal of Adolescent Health* 70, no. 3 (2022): 354, https://doi.org/10.1016/j.jadohealth.2021.12.003.

4 Farzana Akkas, "Youth Suicide Risk Increased Over Past Decade," *The Pew Charitable Trusts,* March 7, 2023, https://www.pewtrusts.org/en/research-and-analysis/articles/2023/03/03/youth-suicide-risk-increased-over-past-decade.

While guns are not the most common method for attempting suicide, they are the most likely to lead to death, and the number of youth gun deaths due to suicide has increased 50% over the past decade. However, while mental illness (specifically depression) likely accounts for increased youth gun *suicide*, studies have found that mental illness rates do not correlate well with gun *homicide* rates.

The factors that predispose an individual to gun homicide are highly complex, as summarized in a 2013 report from the American Psychological Association.[5] These include early childhood experiences of violence, biological and environmental risks in the prenatal and early childhood periods, family factors, and others, all of which interact in complex ways. The report also points out that the number of individuals predisposed to violence is very small. Moreover, few perpetrators of gun violence have overt mental health diagnoses that would predict violence, and conversely, the vast majority of individuals with mental health problems are not prone to violence. All of this suggests that a simple focus on mental health would do little by itself to address interpersonal gun violence.

Social Contributors to Child Gun Deaths

Social factors include both those that might promote gun violence and those that might prevent it. Research has shown that exposure to depictions of violence in media (including mass media, social media, and video games) is correlated with subsequent aggressive

---

5 Dewey Cornell et al., "Gun Violence: Prediction, Prevention, and Policy," *American Psychological Association*, 2013, https://www.apa.org/pubs/reports/gun-violence-prevention.

attitudes and behaviors, though not specifically to gun violence per se.[6] As is often the case in the biopsychosocial model, exposure to media violence likely interacts with individual factors in complex and unpredictable ways. Nevertheless, the weight of evidence suggests that a violent milieu is a contributing factor to gun violence.

It may also be a factor in the minority of child gun deaths that are accidental. Researchers at Ohio State studied 104 children ages 8–12.[7] After randomly viewing movie clips with or without guns, a pair of children (who had both watched the same movie) was taken to a different room with toys and told they could play with any of the toys while they waited. Also in the room was a cabinet with a 9-mm handgun (modified to be unfireable). Overall, 83% of children found the gun, and almost half picked it up. There was no difference between gun-watching and non-gun-watching participants in regard to finding or picking up the gun. But children who had just finished watching a movie containing guns held the gun three times longer and pulled the trigger twenty-two times more often than children who saw the gun-free movie clip. Kids who had watched the movie with guns were also more likely to point the gun at the other child in the room and use threatening language.

6 Huesmann, L. Rowell. 2007. "The Impact of Electronic Media Violence: Scientific Theory and Research." *Journal of Adolescent Health* 41 (6): S6–13. https://doi.org/10.1016/j.jadohealth.2007.09.005.

7 Kelly P. Dillon and Brad J. Bushman, "Effects of Exposure to Gun Violence in Movies on Children's Interest in Real Guns," *The Journal of the American Medical Association Pediatrics* 171, no. 11 (2017): 1057-1062, https://doi.org/10.1001/jamapediatrics.2017.2229.

The regulatory climate is an important social factor in gun injury, and in recent years, that climate has changed, especially since the Heller decision in 2008 in which the Supreme Court affirmed citizens' rights to own firearms even if they're not part of a "militia" as stated in the Second Amendment. As we will discuss more later, research has shown an inverse correlation between the number and strength of gun regulations and the gun injury death rate. From 1991 to 2016, there was an overall increase in state-level regulations, but these were concentrated in only five states, while sixteen states had a net decrease in regulation.[8]

---

8 Sharkey, Patrick, and Megan Kang. 2023. "The Era of Progress on Gun Mortality: State Gun Regulations and Gun Deaths From 1991 to 2016." *Epidemiology* 34 (6): 786–92. https://doi.org/10.1097/ede.0000000000001662.

CHAPTER 4

SUCCESS STORIES

We solve epidemics with medicine, not politics.

—DR. MEGAN RANNEY,
Brown University School of Public Health

It matters that we define child gun violence as a disease and as an epidemic because that gives us a clear path to prevention, to a scientific, evidence-based solution. To understand why we have an epidemic of gun deaths in children, we must understand the causes, beyond a trigger being pulled. Once we understand all the various factors that cause a child to die from a gunshot—the physical, psychological, and social factors—we can then work to prevent these deaths from happening based on research about what interventions are most effective and putting those to use in the greatest possible way.

There are many examples of success in stemming the tide of communicable and non-communicable public health crises. In the mid-1800s, cholera outbreaks were common in much of Europe. They tended to occur in poor neighborhoods. As a result, many people assumed poverty was the cause, specifically that the indifference of the poor to hygiene and the associated dirty and crowded conditions created a miasma, or atmosphere, that produced disease.

In 1854, John Snow, who is now considered the founder of epidemiology, proved that cholera, in fact, came from contaminated water. (It wasn't until the subsequent work of Louis Pasteur and Edward Koch, leading to the germ theory of disease, that the specific cause was determined to be bacteria in the water.) Educating people about the risks of using water sources located near waste (behavioral factor) and eventually water treatment (social factor) then led to the eradication of cholera in developed countries.

In the late twentieth century, when a mysterious immune deficiency arose in certain high-risk populations such as gay men and IV drug users, some people also postulated that it was caused by their lifestyle. Of course, the discovery of the HIV virus debunked this notion. Appropriate preventive measures—education about safe sex practices (behavioral), screening of blood donations and programs for distributing clean needles and condoms (social), and eventually effective retroviral treatments (biological)—led to sharp decreases in the spread of AIDS.

Cholera, tuberculosis, HIV—these and many other infectious diseases that were previously attributed to moral factors—are now recognized as public health issues. Trying to eliminate such ailments by proselytizing among the poor or "curing" homosexuality would be foolhardy at best. Rather, they have been addressed successfully through public health interventions such as water treatment, immunization, and risk education. What were once the most common causes of death in children have been nearly eliminated in the developed world.

It's important to note that some of these successes came even though they were often politically polarizing as well, at least initially. When the AIDS epidemic began, some public officials tried to deny it even existed, while others simply avoided the issue, fearing backlash from social conservatives for tackling what was derided as "the gay disease." Yet Surgeon General Dr. C. Everett Koop, in one of the most conservative administrations in the US in decades, was a key leader in the healthcare system's response.

As with cholera and HIV, some argue that gun violence is a moral issue: guns don't kill people; bad people kill people. Or at best, it's a mental health issue. But it's not, at least not primarily. Nor is it strictly a gun issue. It's a public health issue. And only public health methods, like what we used during the COVID-19 pandemic, will be successful in controlling it.

CHAPTER 5

THE COVID-19 BLUEPRINT

While it is both true and sad (and depressing and infuriating) that gun injury now claims the lives of more kids than anything else, there is another reason to focus attention on the problem now. Gun injury is a bigger health crisis for American kids than before, but frankly, it's been a crisis for a very long time. It's been a crisis we have struggled unsuccessfully to address. I, and many others, have begun to doubt our ability as a nation to deal with a health crisis that often masquerades as a "political" crisis.

The difference now, I think, is COVID-19. COVID-19 showed all of us how to (at least relatively) successfully deal with a public health crisis. It's no longer an abstraction. We know the steps we need to take to ameliorate an epidemic and that those steps must include a combination of medical, behavioral, and policy actions.

A Guide for Gun Safety

Not only do we recognize that gun violence is a public health crisis, especially for kids, and that we have a method, the biopsychosocial model, for addressing such a public health threat, but we also have a recent example of the biopsychosocial public health model in action that we can learn from for protecting kids from gun violence: the COVID-19 pandemic.

Gun violence and COVID-19 are both public health crises; both have become partisan issues. Yet despite the partisanship that crept into efforts to contain COVID-19, healthcare professionals persisted. They applied the biopsychosocial model to COVID-19 just as they would to any other public health crisis, and for the most part, it worked. Their tenacity saved many lives. We can do the same for gun violence.

Because of COVID-19, most of us are familiar with the different parts of the public health model used to control the virus' spread. It became part of our daily lives. People outside the realm of health care might not have defined what they were experiencing with the term "biopsychosocial model," but they were taking a crash course in it just the same.

On the news and in our own lives, we saw that, when it came to the spread of disease, biological, psychological, and social factors mattered. We came to understand how we could become infected with a fast-spreading virus called COVID-19 and what steps we could take to protect ourselves and others.

Applying the biopsychosocial model to COVID-19, to a large extent, worked. The payoff was and continues to be enormous. Research done, behaviors adopted, and policies enacted during COVID-19 saved millions of lives. The vaccine alone has prevented more than eighteen million hospitalizations, three million deaths, and more than $1 trillion in medical costs.[1]

---

1 Meagan C. Fitzpatrick et al., "Two Years of U.S. COVID-19 Vaccines Have Prevented Millions of Hospitalizations and Deaths," *The Commonwealth Fund,* December 13, 2022, https://www.commonwealthfund.org/blog/2022/two-years-covid-vaccines-prevented-millions-deaths-hospitalizations.

Before we apply the biopsychosocial model to the gun crisis, let's explore more about how it was applied to COVID-19. After we review those specifics, we'll be ready to see how the biopsychosocial model can help us reduce the gun violence that threatens our kids' health and lives.

Recall from Chapter 4 that the biopsychosocial model addresses disease from three angles:

- biological (physical)
- psychological (behavioral)
- social (environmental)

Let's look at how each component was applied to contain the COVID-19 pandemic.

Biological

When people first started showing up with a new respiratory illness, doctors didn't know what it was. Pretty quickly, they determined they were dealing with a virus. They examined it through a microscope and sequenced its genome. They started to define its biological, or physical, characteristics and gave it a name. SARS-CoV-2 is the virus that causes the respiratory disease known as COVID-19.

We may never know exactly how, when, or where SARS-CoV-2 infected the first human. But we do know, through the lens of the biopsychosocial model, that SARS-CoV-2 is the biological agent of harm. We know that, when SARS-CoV-2 enters the body of a human being, certain things happen. The virus sparks a chain reaction. The immune system senses the virus and mounts an attack. That interaction between the virus and the immune system is what creates the illness.

So the biological part of the biopsychosocial model shows up in several ways. There's the biology of the virus: what it looks like, what its characteristics are, how it spreads. There's also the physical effect the virus has once it enters the human body. Some people, because of their biological makeup, don't contract the virus despite being exposed to it. Others contract it and have mild to moderate symptoms. Still others, because of their personal biological characteristics (age, sex, underlying disease, etc.), contract the virus and suffer severe symptoms and sometimes death.

Medical care is typically focused largely on addressing the biological aspects of a disease: vaccines for prevention, medications and supportive therapies for managing disease when it occurs. And certainly, these are an important element of dealing with disease on a population scale. But remember, when the COVID-19 pandemic began, there was not yet a vaccine or an effective medication. Supportive care such as mechanical ventilation for severe cases was available, but in the setting of a pandemic, health systems globally became overwhelmed.

So in the early stages, while learning as much as we could about the biology of the virus and its impact on the human body proceeded as quickly as possible, we had to move on to the second and third parts of the biopsychosocial model to address the threat. While our specific knowledge of the SARS-CoV-2 virus was initially limited, we knew enough about respiratory viruses to take steps to control it.

Psychological

As we will see, the three parts of the biopsychosocial model are intertwined. Medications are not useful if people don't seek medical care; masks are not effective if they are not worn; social distancing doesn't work if one's environment doesn't permit it. So first, healthcare workers needed to convince people that the virus was a serious matter. The public needed to understand psychologically what COVID-19 was and that it was an urgent threat; a COVID-19 infection could result in death. Public health professionals disseminated this information often and in many ways. You may have learned about COVID-19 on social media, at your workplace, in the news, or during conversations with family and friends.

When you first heard about COVID-19, you may have shrugged it off, thinking it wouldn't affect you. But when the maps of affected areas started to grow exponentially, when public places, workplaces and borders of countries started shutting down, and when the number of deaths started rising, it was hard not to feel the gravity of what was happening. Once people started understanding the danger the virus posed, our thoughts, emotions, and behaviors changed. Many of us became fearful that we or a loved one would catch the virus. That fear motivated changes in our actions.

This was important because the most effective measures for controlling the spread of COVID-19 and saving lives at the start of the pandemic were, in fact, behavioral measures. This included things like wearing a mask, maintaining physical distance from others, and washing hands far more frequently than most of us normally would.

Before COVID-19, if you saw someone wearing a mask in public, you might have thought that was strange. Soon, covering your face became normal behavior; it was strange if you *didn't* wear a mask. Before COVID-19, it was unusual to see hand sanitizer. Soon, hand sanitizer was available wherever you went.

These were new behaviors for many of us. But most of us quickly got used to them, and that's for a few reasons. First, our mindset, our psychology, had shifted; our fear of catching a potentially deadly disease motivated us to behave in ways we normally wouldn't. Secondly—and this is where the third part of the biopsychosocial model comes in—these new behaviors became socially acceptable and sometimes required by policy.

Social

Attempts to slow the spread of COVID-19 resulted in swift and significant changes in our society. COVID-19 affected our social lives: we canceled major life events like weddings and funerals, while get-togethers with friends and family, even dates, happened virtually or not at all. It changed our society all the way down to how many feet we could safely stand from another person. Shopping and dining became online activities. Some businesses failed, while entirely new ones started up.

There was enormous social pressure to follow these new norms. However, these new behaviors were also reinforced by policy decisions. Schools closed, and businesses were ordered to shut down or restrict their hours and operations. Many state governments ordered citizens not to leave their homes.[2] For example, Hawaii residents who violated their stay-at-home order could be fined $5,000 or face a year in jail.

These social impacts of COVID-19 in turn affected our psychology. Many people suffered from the loss of social interaction, including many children who no longer had direct contact with teachers and couldn't gather in person with friends. And none of us had ever lived through a global pandemic, so some of these measures seemed extreme. But most of us followed them because we wanted to stay safe. And we saw that they worked. When we masked up and social distanced, we could minimize the spread of disease, protect our health, and save lives.

Biopsychosocial Again

As research rapidly progressed, methods of rapid diagnosis and more effective treatments to deal with the physical effects of infection became available, leading to biological approaches to reduce spread and decrease mortality. But these, too, required behavioral and social approaches to advance them. People started to seek out testing when they had symptoms. The government made testing centers and, eventually, home test kits available for free, and testing was required for certain activities such as travel or attending public events.

And then came the vaccine. Its creation and implementation can also be viewed through the biopsychosocial model. The biological is

---

2 Sarah Mervosh, Denise Lu, and Vanessa Swales, "See Which States and Cities Have Told Residents to Stay at Home," *The New York Times*, April 20, 2020, https://www. nytimes.com/interactive/2020/us/coronavirus-stay-at-home-order.html.

the vaccine itself: how it was developed and how it interacts with the human body to minimize a COVID-19 infection. The psychological was educating people about the vaccine, convincing them that it's safe and effective. Once people were on board psychologically, their behavior followed. They made appointments to get the vaccine.

But that didn't happen in all cases; not everyone believes the vaccine is safe, effective, or necessary. That's where the social component of the biopsychosocial model comes back into play. Social policies were enacted to encourage vaccination. The federal government and many health systems mandated that workers be vaccinated. Incentives were created; vaccinated Illinois residents were automatically entered into a $10 million sweepstakes. In some friend and family circles, if you weren't vaccinated for COVID-19, you weren't allowed to socialize in person with the group. There was enormous pressure to get vaccinated.

The Three-Legged Stool

The goal of the biopsychosocial model is controlling disease. Any one part of it alone won't achieve that goal. If we just studied the biological characteristics of COVID-19, that would do nothing to stop its spread. If we created a vaccine but didn't educate people about it or provide opportunities or requirements for people to get it, many fewer people would be vaccinated.

The biopsychosocial model is like a three-legged stool. We need all three legs for it to work. Masks play a role in reducing the spread of COVID-19. The effectiveness depends on the characteristics of the masks (biological/physical) and also on whether they are worn consistently and correctly (psychological/behavioral). Changes in behavior to promote the appropriate use of masks occur through education, social pressures, and policies (social/environmental).

The three components of the biopsychosocial model also don't necessarily appear neatly or in order. They reared their heads at different times throughout the pandemic. Early in the pandemic, there was greater reliance on behavior change in the face of minimal knowledge about the virus and how to attack it biologically. At the same time, there was initially also a higher acceptance of behavioral adaptations and reinforcing policies, but the degree of resistance grew as the pandemic dragged on and treatments and vaccines became available. That resistance led to new policies, albeit variably adapted across different jurisdictions.

A Key Lesson

One of the key lessons from the COVID-19 pandemic is that we need to follow the science to the extent possible. A key corollary to this is that we need to advance the science. Early in the pandemic, we knew little, and some interventions needed to be modified as we learned more.

What was truly remarkable was the breathtaking pace at which the science advanced. It was a matter of mere weeks from when cases of a novel coronavirus infection were first identified to when the genetic sequence of that coronavirus was known. And the time to develop the first effective vaccine was far shorter than had ever been the case before.

While we have a substantial body of knowledge on the physical, behavioral, and social aspects of the pandemic of firearm injury, there is much more we need to learn about which interventions will effectively reduce gun injury and death. As was noted previously, funding for research on gun violence is proportionately far less than for other significant health threats. If we are going to recognize gun violence as a public health crisis and act accordingly, we need to significantly increase the amount of research on it.

The Blueprint Works If You Work It

The important lesson here is that COVID-19 clearly showed us what we need to do to protect ourselves during a public health crisis. We learned that, if we attacked the virus using the biopsychosocial model, we could slow its spread and save lives.

I experienced the pandemic as an ordinary citizen, and I also experienced it as the CEO of a pediatric health system, Children's Minnesota. During the height of COVID-19, we coordinated with other health systems around the state to reinforce important messages about how to stay safe. In the more conservative, rural parts of Minnesota, health systems courageously stayed on message, strongly advocating for public health measures that would minimize COVID-19, even though some residents disagreed with those messages.

Despite the backlash, healthcare professionals persisted—insisting that, yes, you must wear a mask and get vaccinated if you want to save lives. Yes, COVID-19 is a public health issue, not a partisan one. The leader of a health system in rural Minnesota was willing to tell people

COVID-19 is real, to tell employees they had to be vaccinated if they wanted to work there because this wasn't about the partisan politics of vaccines and masks and school closings. It was about public health.

So it struck me when, a couple of years later, this same group of health systems from across Minnesota was crafting another joint statement about another public health crisis: gun violence. The original draft of the statement strongly advocated for policy solutions, but some health systems wanted to back away from that. So we weakened the statement. We ended up calling guns a public health crisis, which is great, but did not advocate for specific action to address it. It occurred to me that we were saying it was a public health crisis, but we were not acting like it. I had seen what it was to act like we were in a public health crisis. I just saw it with COVID-19, and this wasn't it.

If it's a public health problem that's killing our kids, we must treat it as such, follow the same steps we would follow for any other public health problem because they work.

We have the blueprint for solving a public health crisis. While it's still fresh in our minds, let's use it to tackle gun violence the way we tackled COVID-19. If we address gun violence using the same public health model, the same public health tactics, we will see the same results.

CHAPTER 6

HOW DO WE FIX IT?

Many physicians, professional societies, and health systems—in response to recent increases in gun deaths, and mass shootings in particular—have issued a call to recognize gun violence as a public health crisis. But this can't merely be an exercise in raising awareness. If we believe gun violence is a public health crisis, we need to *act* like it is a public health crisis.

When COVID-19 struck, the healthcare community didn't simply issue statements about what a problem it was. We acted. We need to do the same with gun violence. It is long past time to do more than stand idly by and watch the same tragedy replay day after day, month after month, year after year.

As we discussed in Chapter 5, in COVID-19, we have a recent, widely understood plan for containing a health threat. We can take what we've learned about containing COVID-19 and apply it to the gun crisis.

As with COVID-19, that plan is based on the biopsychosocial model of public health, one that recognizes the need to address all three sides of the triad and the interactions between them. It should also be based, as much as possible, on evidence. So let's look at what the evidence tells us works for each side of the triad of gun violence. (For a more thorough review of the evidence, with references, see the Technical Report on Firearm-Related Injuries and Deaths in Children and Youth from the AAP.)[1]

Biological

This is the part of the triad that deals with the physical agent of harm, in this case, the gun and the ammunition. Logic would suggest that eliminating the harmful agent would eliminate the harm, and cross-national epidemiologic studies do show a strong correlation between the number of guns and gun deaths. However, this would undoubtedly be politically and culturally impossible in the United States; furthermore, those same studies also suggest that elimination of guns is not necessary to substantially mitigate the risk.

Earlier we showed that the harm potential for guns and bullets is not uniform for all types and that lethality for both the weapons and the ammunition has increased in recent decades. Measures to limit the more deadly types of guns (e.g., large caliber, semi and fully automatic) and bullets would be expected to lead to fewer injuries and deaths. Numerous studies indeed provide evidence that limiting assault-type weapons reduces gun injury. Unfortunately, there have been few measures to address other gun and bullet characteristics that would allow us to conclude whether such measures would produce the desired public health benefit.

---

1 Lois K. Lee et al., "Firearm-Related Injuries and Deaths in Children and Youth: Injury Prevention and Harm Reduction," *Pediatrics* 150, no. 6 (2022), https://doi.org/10.1542/peds.2022-060070.

Nevertheless, the basic science on the deadliness of certain types of weapons is clear. It's also worth noting that any given weapon tends to be more lethal to younger victims. When comparing school shootings with assault-style weapons, the fatality rate was highest in the youngest victims. Of the school-age children in Sandy Hook, for instance, no child who was shot survived.[2]

Another physical approach is modifying weapons to make it harder for them to cause harm. Safety locks reduce accidental injury. By forcing an additional step prior to firing, they may also serve a 'cooling off' function and lead to a reduction in intentional harm. Mechanisms such as fingerprint detection and other "smart" technology, which prevent the gun from being fired by someone other than the owner, reduce the risk of the gun being stolen or used by a child who comes across the gun. Other modifications make the bullets non-lethal, such as using blunt projectiles or projectiles containing pepper spray.

Safe storage practices are a similar approach. It is important to note that neither a gun nor a bullet is harmful on its own. Rather, it is the gun-bullet system that can deliver harm. Keeping guns and ammunition separate and locked is associated with reduced risk of accidental harm and intentional self-harm. For example, a recent study found that almost one third of youth suicides and accidental deaths could be prevented if adults who have children in their

---

2 Barron, James. 2012. "Children Were All Shot Multiple Times With a Semiautomatic, Officials Say." *The New York Times,* December 15, 2012. https://www.nytimes.com/2012/12/16/nyregion/gunman-kills-20-children-at-school-in-connecticut-28-dead-in-all.html.

homes would safely store their firearms.[3] Safe storage also reduces the risk of theft.

Finally, while eliminating the physical agent may be impossible, reducing it is feasible. The notion of gun buy-back programs has been around since at least the 1990s. The evidence on these programs shows that they do not tend to have a significant impact on community-wide levels of crime in general and gun violence specifically. This appears to be due to their limited scale compared to the massive magnitude of the gun problem. On the other hand, there is anecdotal evidence that they can be a cost-effective means of removing at least some guns from the community.[4]

Psychological

Raising the issue of mental health is a favorite tactic of those who oppose measures to make guns and ammunition safer. As we saw in Chapter 5, the biopsychosocial model shows us that addressing only one leg of the stool is unlikely to be effective in isolation. But those same public health principles tell us we can't ignore the psychological or behavioral side of the triad.

There is widespread recognition of the increased incidence of mental health problems such as depression and anxiety, especially among children and teens. In the 2020s, rates of emergency department visits for youth mental health crises have increased nationally

---

3 Monuteaux, Michael C., Azrael, Deborah, Miller, Matthew, "Association of Increased Safe Household Firearm Storage with Firearm Suicide and Unintentional Death Among US Youth," The Journal of the American Medical Association Pediatrics 173, no. 7 (2019): 657–662 https://www.ncbi.nlm.nih.gov/pmc/articles/PMC6515586/.

4 Brownlee, Chip. 2023. "Gun Buybacks Are Popular, but Do They Work?" The Trace. April 21, 2023. https://www.thetrace.org/2023/04/do-gun-buybacks-work-research-data/.

by around 30%.[5] Equally apparent is that the resources available to address this crisis are woefully inadequate. Wait times for counseling have increased, and access to mental health services along the entire spectrum, from preventive measures to crisis care, has not kept pace with demand.[6]

However, the evidence would suggest that the impact of greater access to mental health services on gun violence would be relatively modest. The vast majority of individuals with mental health problems are nonviolent. Conversely, the vast majority of homicides are committed by people without a mental health problem. Even among mass shooters, who account for only a small percentage of all gun injuries, many have no prior history of mental health concerns. (You could easily argue that anyone who shoots up an elementary school is by definition mentally ill, and most people would agree. The point here is that, in many of those cases, that shooting is the first sign of mental illness, so better mental health services wouldn't have prevented them.)

The impact on suicide would likely be greater, but in many cases, the suicide attempt is the initial manifestation of depression. When that attempt is made with a gun, it is far more likely to lead to death. So broad investment in mental health is certainly desirable but unlikely by itself to substantially reduce the toll of gun violence for our children.

Two more targeted approaches to the behavioral side of the biopsychosocial triad have been shown to be effective. Background checks

5 Loredana Santo et al., "NHSR 191: Emergency Department Visits Related to Mental Health Disorders Among Children and Adolescents, United States, 2018-2021," *National Center for Health Statistics,* no. 191 (2023): 2, https://www.cdc.gov/nchs/data/nhsr/nhsr191.pdf.
6 Aacap. n.d. "Severe Shortage of Child and Adolescent Psychiatrists Illustrated in AACAP Workforce Maps." https://www.aacap.org/aacap/zLatest_News/Severe_Shortage_Child_Adolescent_Psychiatrists_Illustrated_AACAP_Workforce_Maps.aspx.

are designed to keep individuals with a criminal record indicative of violent tendencies from acquiring a gun. Several studies support the effectiveness of background checks in reducing gun injury.[7] So-called red-flag laws, which allow law enforcement to temporarily restrict access to firearms for individuals demonstrating high risk of threat of harm to self or others, are another tailored behavioral approach with supportive evidence behind it.[8]

There have been community-based programs to identify high-risk individuals for a multi-pronged preventive intervention. The Roca program, started in Massachusetts, is one such program that uses behavioral-theory techniques to reduce the risk of enrollees in the program engaging in violent conflict. Independent evaluations have shown moderate evidence that this approach, while relatively resource-intensive, can reduce violent recidivism among participants.

There are also secondary prevention programs where victims of interpersonal violence receive services, including both social supports and behavioral interventions, to reduce the risk of re-injury. Examples include Project Ujima in Milwaukee and Next Step in Minneapolis, which also have evidence of their effectiveness in reducing repeat injury.

Social

The broader environment in which guns and people exist constitutes the third side of the triad. There is evidence that the ubiquity of vio-

---

7 Everytown. n.d. "Background Checks on All Gun Sales | Everytown." https://www.everytown.org/solutions/background-checks/.

8 Everytown. n.d. "Extreme Risk Laws | Everytown." https://www.everytown.org/solutions/extreme-risk-laws/.

lence in general, and guns in particular, in society and especially in the media is a factor contributing to gun injury. It seems too simplistic to say violence in the media causes gun violence in society. After all, gun violence long predates visual media. Rather, regular portrayals of weapons in movies and video games turn a gun into a familiar everyday object that has utility as opposed to an unusual, potentially dangerous object that one should be careful around.

In one intriguing study that supports this notion, researchers randomly showed a group of young children movies either with or without guns.[9] Afterward, those children who had seen the movie with guns were more likely to pick up, play with, and aim a gun they found than the children who had seen the other movie.

Other interventions addressing environmental factors may also reduce gun violence. One is the notion of violence interruption. This involves recruiting community members to identify and intervene in high-risk situations. Examples include Cure Violence in Chicago and Safe Streets in Baltimore.

While there is anecdotal evidence to support these approaches, systematic evidence to date is sparse. Given the widening popularity and geographic spread of these programs, however, they are ripe for study.

As we discussed in Chapter 1, there are long-standing social and economic disparities in our country that have resulted in communities where poverty and hopelessness are rampant, and so is gun violence. Research shows a correlation between poverty and

---

9   Dillon and Bushman, "Effects of Exposure," 1057-1062.

gun violence, and young people who are Black or Latino are disproportionately affected.[10] Every child deserves to grow up in a safe community. Too many kids live in neighborhoods without safe housing and good schools, where jobs and opportunities are scarce and where trust between the police and community members is broken. And addressing these underlying disparities is certainly necessary—that topic is worthy of a book in itself! But lessening economic inequality and systemic racism is not by itself going to fix the problem of gun violence. In following the analogy to COVID-19, it is important and worthwhile to address the comorbid conditions that increase the lethality of COVID-19, but we also needed to deal with COVID-19 itself.

Effective Interventions

We can see that there is a plethora of evidence supporting the effectiveness of a variety of interventions that address each of the three sides of our public health triad of gun injury. How can healthcare professionals and others who want to see a reduction in the number of children dying from gun injury put these into practice?

One approach is to incorporate it into our clinical care. The AAP and others endorse including gun safety as an aspect of anticipatory guidance. This can include safe storage practices, mental health screening, media habits, and asking about guns in the home and in places children visit and then providing evidence-based advice about reducing

---

10 Nicole Kravitz-Wirtz et al., "Inequities in Community Exposure to Deadly Gun Violence by Race/Ethnicity, Poverty, and Neighborhood Disadvantage among Youth in Large US Cities," *Journal of Urban Health* 99, no. 4 (2022): 610-625, https://doi.org/10.1007/s11524-022-00656-0.

these risk factors. Unfortunately, there is limited evidence to support that this approach actually reduces gun injuries or deaths.

Another is direct action. Pediatricians and children's health systems can partner with others to implement interventions such as violence interruption or a gun buy-back. We took this approach at Children's Minnesota. Partnering with several community organizations, we hosted a community health fair including a gun buy-back. We had hoped to get around sixty to eighty guns; we ended up with 119. That's 119 fewer guns in our community, 119 fewer opportunities for a child to be shot to death.

We have also just started participating in the Next Step program I mentioned earlier in this chapter. Here's how it works: when a child or teen comes to one of our hospitals with a gunshot wound, our staff notifies the Next Step staff who come to the hospital for an intervention with the patient and family, connecting them with resources and services they may need while in the hospital. After discharge, Next Step staff follows up with the patient and family, connecting them to resources and services in the community to help prevent the child from getting injured again. As I mentioned, programs like Next Step have been shown to reduce re-injury in kids who are violently assaulted. Next Step is a collaboration with the City of Minneapolis and two Twin Cities health systems, Hennepin Healthcare and North Memorial Hospital.

The approach best supported by the evidence, however, is legislation. Most of the effective approaches to the physical, behavioral, and social factors in the gun violence crisis are amenable to public policy solutions. And the evidence is strong that legislation produces results. When considering both self-inflicted firearm deaths and homicides, several studies have shown that implementation of gun access and safety legislation leads to a reduction in rates and that states with more and stronger firearm access and safety laws have lower rates of firearm death than states with fewer and/or weaker laws.[11] Healthcare professionals who want to see legislation that will protect their patients and their communities need to advocate for it.

At Children's Minnesota, we prioritize gun violence prevention in our advocacy work with city and state officials. That means submitting written and in-person testimony to legislative committees. It means speaking out in other ways, too, to persuade lawmakers and the general public through blogs, public statements, newspaper opinion pieces, and working with the news media to get coverage on the effects gun violence has on our children.

It's also important that we come together whenever possible. We in health care share a unique perspective on this public health crisis. At Children's Minnesota, we have a front-row seat to how gun violence impacts children and families and our communities at large, so we have joined a national coalition of hospitals working to reduce gun injury and death in our kids.[12] We have also joined a coalition of Minnesota hospitals working to do the same.

Forging alliances, followed by concrete action, is important. We are stronger together.

---

11 Everytown for Gun Safety Support Fund. 2024. "Gun Safety Policies Save Lives." Everytown Research & Policy. February 23, 2024. https://everytownresearch.org/rankings/.

12 "13 Kids Are Killed by Guns Every Day." n.d. https://www.hospitalsunited.com/.

CHAPTER 7

PEDIATRICIANS IN ACTION

Every year, Gallup asks Americans which professionals they trust most. Medical doctors consistently rank near the top. So do nurses. Even cutting across political lines—Republicans, Democrats, and Independents—all consider nurses and doctors to be among our country's most trustworthy professionals.[1]

Their words—and their actions—matter to people.

Pediatricians are dedicated to the wellness of their young patients. We study the latest treatments, search for cures, and most of all, we work to prevent those things that threaten the health of children.

That is precisely why pediatricians, and health care professionals in general, are well suited to deliver a potentially controversial message, a message that is often interpreted as partisan when it really is about preventing children from falling victim to the number one threat to their lives.

The message is this: guns are a public health crisis for our children. As such, we are approaching this issue as we would any public

1 Lydia Saad, "U.S. Ethics Ratings Rise for Medical Workers and Teachers," *Gallup,* December 22, 2020, https://news.gallup.com/poll/328136/ethics-ratings-rise-medical-workers-teachers.aspx.

health issue. We are focusing on prevention. And there are things we can do both in the clinical setting and outside it to be advocates for our patients.

Outside the Doctor's Office

The AAP has been sounding the alarm about guns as a public health threat to children for at least thirty years. After all, many pediatricians have a front-row seat. In 2022, more than 300 of them submitted personal statements to Congress on the impact of gun violence in their hospitals, their communities, and their personal lives.

Pediatricians across the country have been advocating for solutions for decades. The AAP wants Congress to enact common-sense gun legislation that strengthens background checks, encourages safe firearm storage, bans assault weapons, and addresses firearm trafficking among other things.

I think the AAP is a very strong and effective advocate for kids' health initiatives. This is the primary reason I have belonged to the AAP for thirty years. As an organization, they are a respected voice when it comes to advocating for kids' health issues.

But pediatricians as individuals don't always see it as their role to advocate for the changes the AAP is pushing for. And some pro-gun advocates have criticized physicians and other health professionals who do speak out, telling them to "stay in your lane." But I feel like it is part of our job as pediatricians to champion change that could save children's lives. When it comes specifically to the issue of guns, which are now the leading cause of death for children, that is most definitely in our lane. Yet people can be uncomfortable because it's often characterized as a political issue. This is where I think it's helpful to frame it as a public health issue. You're not advocating on a political issue; you're advocating on a public health issue that affects the health of your patients.

The AAP is doing its part—leading the charge, being vocal, advocating for widespread policy change. And some individual pediatricians are, too. That's the picture outside the doctor's office. What's being done inside the doctor's office to prevent gun violence against children?

Inside the Doctor's Office

A core part of pediatrics as a specialty is emphasizing prevention. We give vaccines, we give anticipatory guidance, and we help kids and parents understand how to prevent injuries and illnesses.

As pediatricians, we're very strongly inculcated throughout our training and our careers on the importance of prevention. The idea is that, if there's a health issue, if there is something that can prevent it, it is certainly within our bailiwick to do so. And now that we have this very stark reminder that, of all the things we're trying to prevent, gun violence is the number one cause of death for kids, prevention is important.

We might say, well, we can't prevent everything. We give vaccines to prevent illness. We don't prevent every case of it, but it helps. We advise parents on car seat and seatbelt safety. We can't force them to use car seats or seatbelts, but we still encourage it. We work toward prevention, even if we don't think it's always perfectly effective. Even if it's not totally within our control as medical professionals, we give preventive advice.

There is no law, federal or state, prohibiting pediatricians from discussing gun safety with patients and their families (although some have been proposed). If we want to focus our prevention efforts, we should focus on the biggest threats facing kids, and today, that would be gun violence.

Supporting Pediatricians as Advocates

A growing number of pediatricians believe it's their role to discuss gun violence prevention with their patients and families. In the 2019 Periodic Survey of Fellows by the AAP, the vast majority of pediatricians surveyed, 92%, agree that violence prevention should be a priority for pediatricians. Over 90% agree that discussions of gun safety should be part of routine preventive care.[2]

Yet it doesn't actually happen routinely. According to the Kaiser Family Foundation survey, only 26% of parents of children under eighteen say their healthcare provider talked with them about guns in the home.[3] Why this disconnect? Among the contributing factors revealed in an earlier survey of pediatricians, 30% reported being uncomfortable having those conversations, 36% said their patient families resented being asked about guns, and 80% said they simply did not have time.[4]

---

2 "Gun Safety and Injury Prevention," *American Academy of Pediatrics,* June 20, 2023, https://www.aap.org/en/patient-care/gun-safety-and-injury-prevention/.

3 Schumacher et al., "Americans' Experience."

4 "Survey: Gun violence prevention a big issue for most pediatricians," *American Academy of Pediatrics News,* August 10, 2016, https://publications.aap.org/aapnews/news/14151/Survey-Gun-violence-prevention-a-big-issue-for.

Pediatricians have direct contact with patients; they're on the front lines, in exam rooms with patients and families, especially during well checks. What more can be done to ease the path for conversations about gun violence prevention? Lack of recent experience with a clinical problem and lack of formal training may reduce a provider's comfort with providing anticipatory guidance.

While most pediatric residents (69%) surveyed in 2019 reported having had experience treating a patient with a firearm injury during their training, only 14% of practicing pediatricians reported treating or consulting on a gun injury in the prior year.[5] In addition, pediatric trainees in one recent study reported a lack of knowledge about how to effectively counsel families on safe storage and other aspects of firearm safety.[6] Given the public health importance of gun injury for children, the subject should be given more emphasis in both graduate medical education and continuing medical education to ensure pediatricians have the skills they need.

We also know that even when they want to discuss gun injury prevention with families, providers simply do not have enough time. Pediatricians have a long list of health threats to review with patients during well checks. Preventive visits are getting shorter, and the number of things pediatricians are supposed to give guidance on is getting longer. But surely there's time to cover the threat that's taking more lives than any other? Of course, that's easier said than done.

The economics of children's health care make it unlikely that preventive visits are going to get dramatically more expansive. Novel

---

5 "Gun Safety."
6 Katherine Hoops and Cassandra Crifasi, "Pediatric resident firearm-related anticipatory guidance: Why are we still not talking about guns?", *Preventative Medicine* 124 (2019): 29-32, https://doi.org/10.1016/j.ypmed.2019.04.020.

approaches to anticipatory guidance need to be developed, and they need to be researched to evaluate whether they work, specifically for the issue of firearm safety. Pediatricians need to continue to advocate to ensure that their right to provide counseling on any health topic, including guns, is not restricted by state law, as has been attempted or proposed in several states. If providers are forced to pick and choose which health risks they are going to focus on in their limited time, they need to be aware of how significant the health risk is from gun injury.

CHAPTER 8

CONCLUSION

When you get right down to it, the solution to the gun crisis facing our kids is relatively simple. It requires a slight shift in our thinking: defining gun violence as a public health crisis since it is now the number one threat to our kids' lives and then combating this public health crisis like we would any other, through a series of steps, the same steps used to reign in COVID-19 and a host of other public health threats.

COVID-19 forced us to re-learn how to deal with a massive, debilitating public health crisis. At the same time, guns became the primary killer of kids in our country. The confluence of those two events gives us a rare opportunity to use our COVID-19 public health crisis knowledge—and the courage to pursue it—to go after another insidious public health threat. There's nothing magic about the solution. It's genius in its simplicity.

But simple doesn't mean easy. Gun violence has so far proven to be an intractable issue. But we do have reasons for hope.

First, we have a moral imperative. We are talking about saving children's lives. Nobody wants to see children die, especially from an entirely preventable cause.

Second, we have the will to accomplish this. We feel it and see it every time children are killed by guns, especially after a mass shooting like Uvalde, Parkland, or Sandy Hook.

But our collective will to combat gun violence comes in fits and starts. When I tell people that guns are the number one killer of kids, that never fails to grab somebody's attention. When there's a mass shooting, the camera captures everybody's attention, but then it fades away. That's a reason to not be necessarily hopeful. If we didn't do it after Uvalde, Parkland, or Sandy Hook, what makes us think we can ever solve this public health crisis? Defining gun violence as a partisan issue leads to hopelessness, throwing our hands in the air in helplessness and frustration. Defining it as a health issue gives us the sustained motivation and resolve to address it like we have so many other health crises.

I know we have the will because I saw it with COVID-19. I've seen it with other health threats that hurt children. If it's tainted food or water, we take measures. If it's lead-tainted toys or jewelry, we take measures. If it's unsafe cribs or furniture, we take measures. How is a gun any different? They're not made specifically for kids, but they are dangerous objects finding their way into the hands of kids or being used against kids. So maybe the more apt analogy is child-proof medicine bottles. Kids were able to open them and swallow harmful pills, so we took measures. Now every bottle containing pills is child-proof. Or there are laundry/dishwasher pods. They are not made for children but were finding their way into the hands of kids. So we took measures.

Our country has a long inspiring history of eradicating health threats to children. Many of the great public health achievements of the twentieth century were the treatment of major causes of death for children. All of these threats have been greatly reduced by using public health model interventions and interruptions. Let's make one of this century's great public health achievements the reduction of gun deaths among children and all of our citizens. It is not a puzzle like cancer. Do we need more research? Yes, but we have a clear road map in the public health triad to help us save lives. This is in our reach. Within our power. Let's do it.

Another reason for hope: in the spring of 2022, Congress finally did pass some federal gun legislation. It is by no means perfect. But shortly before it passed, I and many others would have said there's no way we're getting a gun bill. It's not going to happen. But it happened. (Actually, I did say it. I was glad to be proven wrong.) And in my own state of Minnesota, some meaningful legislation including expanded background checks and a "red-flag" law were enacted and signed in 2023. It is still highly partisan and highly divisive. It is something we've been grappling with for so long, and we've made a little progress. It may not be enough yet, but I'll take any bits of progress I can get.

Are we okay with children dying being the collateral of our gun culture? I don't hate guns. I'm not trying to take them away. It is possible to have a society where guns are legal yet safe. Finland and Canada have similar levels of gun ownership as the US, but death rates are a fraction of ours. It will take legislation and education, both key pillars of successful public health strategies. And those of us who advocate for kids need to help with both.

There is a better way. As we have seen, so many deaths and so much trauma can be prevented by approaching gun violence as we do any other threat to our children's health.

What can you do? The first step was reading this book, understanding the magnitude of the problem for our children, and learning a new way to approach the issue that avoids partisan pitfalls. Keeping the focus on kids' health is key. All political parties, all people, can get behind that.

Talk to people about this public health perspective on the gun issue. Educate them. Share your copy of the book. Talk to friends, family, and everyone in your inner circle.

Branch out from there. If you have children, talk to their pediatrician. Talk to your political representatives. Write them a letter, call them, and schedule a meeting. Refer them to the book or recap it for them. Demand change. Hold them accountable.

If you are a pediatrician or health care worker, talk to your patients. Ask them if there's a gun in their home. Is it locked? Is the ammunition also locked and stored separately?

Consider the issue of guns at the ballot box. Vote for candidates who support these common-sense solutions to gun violence.

It's easy to get discouraged. If parents who've lost kids at Uvalde, Parkland, and Sandy Hook can't make a change, who can? That shows us how intractable the issue has been. But we are living in a new world now. We have a single shocking statistic. Guns are the number one killer of kids. We have lived through COVID-19 and experienced firsthand how to handle a public health crisis, even one that becomes partisan. We know how effective the public health model can be if we follow it.

Let's apply it to the biggest threat of all to our children's lives. It will take all of us. Doctors, nurses, parents, teachers, policymakers, all Americans who care about children and want them to live long healthy lives, free from the mental and physical toll of gun violence.

It starts with each of us making the choice to get on board. It starts with you.

Won't you join us?

AFTERWORD

The average American school bus carries seventy-two children. Imagine if every six days, on a particular section of highway, a school bus crashed and killed every single child on board. Imagine if this went on for a year. Parents, politicians, and the community would be infuriated about why these horrible crashes were happening and demand that something be done to prevent them.

Studies of that section of road, the school buses, the drivers, and a host of other interventions would likely ensue. This crisis of bus crashes that are killing children would be addressed. Sadly, as a society, we have been unable to act with the necessary urgency when a similar number of children are being killed each year by firearms.

Most of these deaths are due to homicide and suicide. African-American and American Indian children bear a disproportionate brunt of these firearm-related deaths. Indeed, African-American teens aged 15–19 are over four times more likely to die from homicide than White youth. In 2022, for the first time, suicide rates for Black children exceeded those for White children. The reasons are complex and myriad but are rooted in poverty and environmental and systemic racism. These limit the opportunities for children to grow up in healthy, violence-free environments. Addressing these conditions is vital to help decrease our youth's exposure to firearm-related injuries and deaths.

In this book, Dr. Gorelick highlights the public health crisis that firearm-related injuries and fatalities constitute. While we comprise less than 5% of the world's population, Americans collectively own about 45% of all privately held firearms in the world. There are more guns than people in this country. For every 100 people, there are more than 120 guns. There are multiple reasons for gun ownership, including sport, hunting, self-protection, and collection. However, guns in the home pose a clear threat to individuals living in that household despite protection being the most common reason that individuals own guns. For every self-defense or justifiable homicide, forty-three individuals in the home die due to firearms, primarily by suicide.

Dr. Gorelick's call to action is timely. An all-hands-on-deck approach must be employed to solve this problem. This includes collaboration among different groups that may not always work together, including public health experts, legislators, law enforcement, youth services, schools, churches, neighborhood groups, and each one of us individually. This work will include reducing poverty and transforming impoverished communities into greener, safer spaces. That will begin to address the impact of environmental and structural racism that has led to the disproportionate impact of firearms in these communities.

This work will also involve programs to reduce community violence, research on firearm injury reduction, programs to address mental health, and targeted legislative actions to reduce firearm-related injuries. I applaud Dr. Gorelick for this work and join him in urging us all to work toward addressing this public health emergency with the urgency it deserves.

Andrew W. Kiragu, MD, FAAP, FCCM

Associate Professor of Pediatrics, University of Minnesota

Associate Chief of Critical Care, Children's Minnesota

Made in the USA
Middletown, DE
07 August 2024

58708407R00059